WATSU THERAPY EXPLAINED

Essential Guide To Unlocking The Healing Benefits Of Aquatic Bodywork For Stress Relief, Pain Management, And Improved Wellbeing

DR. MELISSA STOTLER

Copyright © 2023 by Dr. Melissa Stotler

Disclaimer:

The data in this book, "Acupuncture Therapy Simplified," is solely meant to be informative and instructional.

This book is not intended to replace expert medical advice, diagnosis, or care. No medical, health, or other professional services are offered by the author, publisher, or any affiliated parties

Individual outcomes may differ in the practice of these therapies, which entail a variety of approaches and methodologies.

 A one-on-one session with a trained or certified healthcare professional is still preferable. It is best to consult a trained healthcare provider before making any decisions regarding your health.

The author of this book is not affiliated with any specific website, product, or organization related to any of these therapies.

All reasonable measures have been taken by the author and publisher to guarantee the authenticity and dependability of the material contained in this book.

Contents

Watsu Therapy Explained offers an in-depth exploration of a unique and powerful form of aquatic bodywork that has garnered global recognition for its profound therapeutic benefits. This book delves into the history and origins of Watsu therapy, tracing its development from its inception to its modern-day applications. Readers will be introduced to the key figures who pioneered this therapeutic approach and learn how Watsu has evolved, expanding its influence worldwide. The comprehensive coverage of Watsu's history underscores its significance and the impact it has had on holistic healing practices across cultures.

Understanding the basics of Watsu therapy is essential for both practitioners and clients. The book meticulously outlines the core concepts and fundamental principles that form the foundation of Watsu therapy. It highlights the unique role water plays in enhancing the therapeutic experience, allowing for greater relaxation and mobility. The therapist's responsibilities and techniques are thoroughly explained, providing insights into what clients can expect during a session. Emphasis is placed on safety measures to ensure a secure and effective therapy experience. This section is crucial for demystifying the process and setting clear expectations for anyone new to Watsu.

The techniques and methods employed in Watsu therapy are diverse and adaptable. The book presents a detailed guide to basic and advanced Watsu movements and practices, including breathing and relaxation techniques that enhance the overall effectiveness of the therapy. Readers will learn about proper positioning and support techniques, as well as how to customize therapy to meet individual needs. This practical information is invaluable for practitioners seeking to refine their skills and for clients who wish to understand the intricacies of the therapy they receive.

Watsu therapy offers a multitude of benefits, both physical and emotional. The book explores the relief from pain and improved mobility that many clients experience, as well as the mental and emotional benefits such as stress reduction and emotional healing. Enhanced well-being and quality of life are common outcomes of Watsu therapy, supported by real-life case studies that illustrate successful results. The long-term effects of Watsu are also discussed, highlighting its potential to contribute to sustained health and wellness.

Preparation is key to maximizing the benefits of a Watsu therapy session. The book provides practical pre-session guidelines, including advice on appropriate attire and setting realistic expectations. Effective communication with the therapist is emphasized, ensuring that clients' needs and concerns are addressed. Post-session care tips are also included to help clients continue to reap the benefits of their therapy after leaving the water. This section is designed to empower clients with the knowledge they need to fully engage in and benefit from their Watsu therapy experience.

Watsu therapy can be particularly beneficial for specific conditions. The book discusses how Watsu can assist in managing chronic pain, reducing stress and anxiety, and aiding in physical rehabilitation. It also covers safe practices and benefits for pregnant individuals and adaptations for elderly clients. This targeted information makes the book a valuable resource for individuals with specific therapeutic needs and for practitioners seeking to expand their expertise in these areas.

Addressing common concerns and misconceptions is vital for fostering a clear understanding of Watsu therapy. The book tackles safety concerns, effectiveness doubts, and misunderstandings about water therapy. It also discusses the costs and accessibility of Watsu therapy, guiding finding affordable options.

Tips for choosing a skilled Watsu therapist are included, ensuring that clients can make informed decisions about their care. This candid approach helps to build trust and confidence in the therapy.

The FAQs section answers common questions about Watsu therapy, offering practical advice on what to expect in the first session, how often therapy should be scheduled, potential side effects, and integrating Watsu with other treatments. This section serves as a quick reference guide for both newcomers and seasoned clients, providing clear and concise information on frequently asked questions. Additionally, the book concludes with resources and further reading, directing readers to recommended books, articles, online resources, professional organizations, and opportunities for hands-on learning and certification. This final section encourages continued learning and engagement with the Watsu therapy community, making the book a comprehensive and essential guide for anyone interested in this transformative form of therapy.

CHAPTER ONE

HISTORY AND ORIGINS OF WATSU THERAPY

Foundations Of Watsu: The Origins And Development Of Watsu Therapy

Watsu therapy, an innovative form of bodywork performed in warm water, originated in the early 1980s.

The concept was pioneered by Harold Dull, who was deeply influenced by his studies in Zen Shiatsu.

Combining the principles of Shiatsu with the unique properties of water, Dull created a therapeutic technique that enhances relaxation and promotes healing.

The name "Watsu" is a blend of "water" and "Shiatsu," reflecting its roots in traditional

Japanese massage techniques and its aquatic setting.

Key Figures: Important Individuals Who Contributed to Its Development

Harold Dull stands as the pivotal figure in the creation and dissemination of Watsu therapy. His journey began in Japan, where he studied Zen Shiatsu under the guidance of Shizuto Masunaga.

Bringing these techniques back to the United States, Dull experimented with applying Shiatsu in a warm water pool, finding that the buoyancy of water allowed for greater freedom of movement and deeper relaxation for clients.

Other significant contributors include practitioners and instructors who have helped refine the techniques and expand the practice worldwide, ensuring that Dull's vision continued to evolve.

Evolution Over Time: How Watsu Has Evolved And Expanded

Since its inception, Watsu therapy has undergone significant evolution. Initially focused on the core principles of Zen Shiatsu, the practice has integrated various elements from other bodywork and aquatic therapies.

This evolution has allowed Watsu to address a broader range of physical and emotional conditions.

Techniques have been adapted to include more fluid and dynamic movements, leveraging the resistance and support provided by water.

Training programs and certification processes have also been established to maintain high standards among practitioners, fostering a professional and consistent approach to Watsu therapy.

Global Influence: How Watsu Has Spread Worldwide

Watsu therapy has experienced widespread adoption across the globe. From its beginnings in the United States, the practice quickly spread to Europe, Asia, and beyond.

This global reach has been facilitated by a network of dedicated practitioners and instructors who offer workshops and training sessions internationally.

As more people experience the benefits of Watsu, its popularity continues to grow. The therapy has been incorporated into various health and wellness programs, from rehabilitation centers to luxury spas, making it accessible to a diverse range of clients.

Modern Applications: Contemporary Uses And Practices Of Watsu Therapy

In contemporary settings, Watsu therapy is utilized for a myriad of applications. It is particularly effective in managing chronic pain, reducing stress, and promoting physical rehabilitation.

The gentle movements and warm water environment provide an ideal setting for individuals with mobility issues, allowing for exercise and stretching with minimal strain.

Additionally, Watsu is employed in mental health treatment, helping to alleviate symptoms of anxiety and depression through its profound relaxation effects.

The practice is also popular among athletes for recovery and performance enhancement, and it is increasingly integrated into prenatal care to support expectant mothers.

As the understanding of its benefits expands, Watsu therapy continues to be a versatile and valuable tool in the realm of holistic health.

CHAPTER TWO

UNDERSTANDING THE BASICS OF WATSU THERAPY

Watsu therapy, a blend of water and shiatsu, originated in Japan and has become a sought-after form of bodywork worldwide.

This therapeutic technique takes place in warm water, typically around 35°C (95°F), and combines elements of massage, joint mobilization, muscle stretching, and dance. The warmth of the water promotes relaxation, while the buoyancy aids in gentle stretching and movement.

Watsu sessions are typically conducted in a private or semi-private pool where the client floats while the therapist supports and maneuvers their body. This unique environment allows for a deep state of relaxation, often described as a meditative or trance-like experience. Watsu therapy can help alleviate various physical and emotional conditions, making it a versatile and holistic approach to health and well-being.

Core Concepts: Fundamental Principles Of Watsu Therapy

The core principles of Watsu therapy revolve around trust, relaxation, and the therapeutic properties of warm water. One of the fundamental concepts is buoyancy, which reduces the effects of gravity, allowing for more effortless movements and stretches. This principle facilitates a range of motion that is often unachievable on land.

Another key principle is presence and attunement. The therapist must be fully present and attuned to the client's needs, responding to subtle cues and ensuring the movements are both therapeutic and comforting. The flow and rhythm of the movements are essential, mimicking the gentle ebb and flow of water, creating a soothing and continuous motion.

Breath synchronization is also a vital aspect. Both the client and therapist coordinate their breathing to enhance relaxation and promote a deeper connection. This synchronized breathing helps the client release tension and surrender to the therapeutic process.

The Role Of Water: How Water Enhances The Therapy

Water plays a crucial role in Watsu therapy, offering a unique environment that amplifies the benefits of traditional bodywork.

The warmth of the water aids in relaxing muscles, reducing pain, and increasing blood flow. This thermal effect helps in easing muscle stiffness and promotes a state of calmness and relaxation.

Buoyancy is another significant factor. It allows the body to float, reducing the impact of gravity and enabling the therapist to perform stretches and movements with less resistance. This buoyant environment supports the body, relieving stress on joints and facilitating a broader range of motion.

The hydrostatic pressure of water also contributes to the therapy. This pressure can help reduce swelling, improve circulation, and enhance the lymphatic system's function.

The gentle resistance of water also aids in muscle strengthening and conditioning without the strain experienced on land.

Therapist's Role: The Therapist's Responsibilities And Techniques

The therapist's role in Watsu therapy is multifaceted, combining technical skill with deep empathy and attentiveness. One of their primary responsibilities is to create a safe and supportive environment. This includes maintaining the proper water temperature and ensuring the pool area is clean and free of hazards.

Therapists must be proficient in various techniques, including gentle stretching, joint mobilization, and acupressure.

They use their hands, arms, and sometimes their entire body to support and move the client through the water.

Techniques such as cradling, rocking, and swaying are commonly used to induce relaxation and therapeutic benefits.

Communication and empathy are crucial. The therapist must constantly gauge the client's comfort and adjust techniques accordingly.

This involves verbal communication as well as being sensitive to non-verbal cues. Building trust is essential, as clients need to feel safe and supported to fully relax and benefit from the therapy.

Client Experience: What Clients Should Expect During A Session

Clients embarking on their first Watsu therapy session can expect a deeply relaxing and often transformative experience. Initial consultation is usually conducted to discuss any specific issues or goals and to ensure the client feels comfortable and informed about the process.

During the session, clients are typically instructed to wear a swimsuit and may be provided with additional flotation devices if needed.

The therapist will gently guide the client into the warm water and begin with gentle holding and cradling techniques.

The client will experience a series of movements, stretches, and massages, all performed in a fluid and continuous motion.

The sensation of weightlessness is a unique aspect of Watsu therapy, allowing clients to experience a profound sense of freedom and relaxation.

Many clients report feeling as though they are in a dream-like state, floating effortlessly as the therapist moves them through the water.

Safety Measures: Ensuring Safety During Therapy

Safety is paramount in Watsu therapy, and several measures are in place to ensure a secure and beneficial experience for the client. The therapist is trained to maintain optimal water temperature and quality, ensuring the environment is conducive to relaxation and therapeutic benefits.

Before the session begins, the therapist will conduct a thorough assessment to identify any potential risks or contraindications. Clients with certain medical conditions may require modifications or alternative therapies to ensure their safety.

Continuous monitoring during the session is essential. The therapist remains in close contact with the client, adjusting techniques and support as needed to ensure comfort and safety. Emergency protocols are also established, with therapists trained in water safety and first aid.

By adhering to these safety measures, Watsu therapy can be a profoundly relaxing and healing experience, allowing clients to reap the full benefits of this unique form of bodywork.

CHAPTER THREE

TECHNIQUES AND METHODS IN WATSU THERAPY

Basic Techniques: Fundamental Watsu Movements And Practices

In Watsu therapy, the basic techniques form the foundation of the practice. These fundamental movements are designed to utilize the buoyancy and resistance of water to facilitate a gentle, flowing motion. Practitioners often begin by cradling the recipient in the water, supporting their head and lower back to create a sense of safety and trust.

The movements typically include gentle rocking, stretching, and rotating the body in different directions to release tension and improve flexibility.

A key technique in Watsu is the "water breath dance," where the practitioner synchronizes their movements with the recipient's breathing. This helps to deepen the relaxation response and enhance the therapeutic benefits of the session. Another essential practice is the "snake" movement, where the practitioner gently moves the recipient's arms and legs in a sinuous, wave-like motion to encourage spinal flexibility and alignment.

Breathing And Relaxation: Techniques To Enhance Relaxation And Effectiveness

Breathing and relaxation are central to Watsu therapy, as they help to maximize the therapeutic effects. Practitioners guide recipients in using deep, diaphragmatic breathing to promote relaxation and reduce stress.

This type of breathing involves inhaling deeply through the nose, allowing the abdomen to expand, and exhaling slowly through the mouth.

To enhance relaxation, sessions often begin with guided breathing exercises. The practitioner may instruct the recipient to close their eyes, focus on their breath, and let go of any tension with each exhale. This creates a meditative state that facilitates the body's natural healing processes.

Additionally, the warm water itself plays a crucial role in relaxation. The buoyancy of the water reduces the effects of gravity, allowing muscles to release and joints to decompress. The warm temperature helps to dilate blood vessels, improving circulation and promoting a sense of calm.

Support And Alignment: Proper Positioning And Support Techniques

Proper support and alignment are vital components of Watsu therapy to ensure safety and effectiveness. The practitioner must maintain a secure hold on the recipient while allowing for fluid movement.

 Typically, the practitioner supports the recipient's head and lower back, ensuring their ears remain above water to prevent discomfort.

Alignment techniques involve gently adjusting the recipient's posture to promote optimal body mechanics and prevent strain. For example, during stretches, the practitioner may adjust the recipient's spine to maintain a neutral alignment, supporting the natural curves of the back.

Support also extends to the psychological aspect of therapy. Practitioners create a nurturing environment, offering verbal reassurance and maintaining a calm demeanor to help recipients feel secure and relaxed. This holistic approach ensures that both physical and emotional needs are addressed.

Advanced Techniques: More Complex Movements And Their Benefits

Advanced Watsu techniques build on the foundational practices, incorporating more complex movements to target specific therapeutic goals.

These techniques often require a higher level of skill and experience from the practitioner. One such technique is the "spiral," where the practitioner guides the recipient's body in a continuous, spiraling motion. This movement helps to release deep-seated tension and improve spinal flexibility.

Another advanced technique is the "dolphin," where the practitioner supports the recipient's body in a horizontal position and moves it in a flowing, wave-like pattern. This technique can enhance proprioception, the body's ability to sense its position in space and improve coordination.

Advanced Watsu movements can also involve dynamic stretching and joint mobilization. For example, the practitioner may perform passive range-of-motion exercises to increase joint flexibility and reduce stiffness.

These techniques are particularly beneficial for individuals with chronic pain or mobility issues, as they help to improve function and alleviate discomfort.

Customizing Therapy: Adapting Techniques To Individual Needs

Customizing Watsu therapy to meet individual needs is essential for achieving optimal outcomes. Practitioners assess each recipient's unique physical and emotional conditions and tailor the session accordingly.

For example, individuals with limited mobility may benefit from gentle, supportive movements that focus on pain relief and relaxation, while athletes may require more dynamic stretches to enhance performance and recovery.

The practitioner also takes into account the recipient's preferences and comfort levels. Communication is key; practitioners often check in with recipients throughout the session to ensure they are comfortable and to make any necessary adjustments.

Customization extends to the duration and intensity of the session. Some individuals may benefit from shorter, more frequent sessions, while others may prefer longer, less frequent sessions.

By adapting the therapy to each person's specific needs, practitioners can provide a more effective and personalized therapeutic experience.

CHAPTER FOUR

BENEFITS OF WATSU THERAPY

Physical Health Benefits: Relief From Pain And Improved Mobility

Watsu therapy offers substantial physical health benefits, particularly in relieving pain and enhancing mobility. This unique form of aquatic bodywork involves a practitioner gently cradling, stretching, and massaging a person in warm water. The buoyancy of the water reduces the gravitational pull on the body, which can significantly alleviate joint and muscle pain. The warm water itself also has a soothing effect, which helps to relax tight muscles and reduce inflammation.

One of the key physical benefits is the improvement in mobility. The water environment supports the body, allowing for a greater range of motion than would be possible on land. This is particularly beneficial for individuals with conditions such as arthritis, and fibromyalgia, or those recovering from surgery or injury. The gentle stretches and movements performed during a Watsu session can enhance flexibility and increase circulation, promoting healing and reducing stiffness. Patients often report a significant reduction in pain and an increased ability to perform daily activities with ease after just a few sessions.

Mental And Emotional Benefits: Stress Reduction And Emotional Healing

Beyond the physical advantages, Watsu therapy is renowned for its profound mental and emotional benefits. The combination of warm water and gentle, rhythmic movements creates a deeply relaxing environment that can significantly reduce stress and anxiety. The therapy session often involves elements of mindfulness and breathwork, which help to calm the mind and promote a sense of inner peace.

The emotional healing aspect of Watsu therapy cannot be overstated. The nurturing environment of the water, combined with the therapist's supportive presence, allows individuals to let go of emotional tension and past traumas.

Many participants report experiencing deep emotional releases during sessions, often feeling a sense of being held and supported in a way that fosters emotional healing.

This can lead to improved mood, better sleep, and an overall sense of well-being. The safe, tranquil setting provides a unique opportunity for individuals to connect with their emotions and work through psychological barriers in a supportive, non-judgmental space.

Enhanced Well-Being: Overall Improvements In Quality Of Life

Watsu therapy's holistic approach contributes to enhanced overall well-being and quality of life. The combined physical, mental, and emotional benefits lead to a comprehensive improvement in how individuals feel and function daily. Regular sessions can result in reduced chronic pain, increased physical mobility, and a more relaxed and positive mental state.

Participants often find that their quality of life improves significantly as they become more capable of engaging in physical activities and enjoy better mental health. This improved state of well-being can enhance relationships, increase productivity, and foster a more positive outlook on life. The therapy's ability to address both physical ailments and emotional challenges makes it a powerful tool for comprehensive health improvement.

Case Studies: Real-Life Examples Of Successful Outcomes

Numerous case studies highlight the effectiveness of Watsu therapy. For instance, a study involving individuals with chronic back pain demonstrated significant pain reduction and improved functional mobility after a series of Watsu sessions. Participants reported not only physical relief but also a sense of emotional release and improved mental health.

Another case involved a patient recovering from a stroke, who experienced marked improvements in balance, coordination, and overall mobility. The supportive water environment allowed for safe and effective rehabilitation, facilitating movements that would have been difficult on land.

These real-life examples underscore the multifaceted benefits of Watsu therapy. The positive outcomes reported by participants across various conditions and demographics illustrate the therapy's versatility and effectiveness. Whether dealing with chronic pain, emotional trauma, or rehabilitation, Watsu offers a supportive, nurturing approach to healing and recovery.

Long-Term Effects: How Watsu Can Contribute To Long-Term Health

The long-term effects of Watsu therapy are equally compelling. Consistent participation in Watsu sessions can lead to sustained improvements in physical health, emotional stability, and overall quality of life. The gentle, non-invasive nature of the therapy makes it suitable for long-term use, providing continuous support for chronic conditions and ongoing emotional challenges.

Over time, the cumulative benefits of regular Watsu therapy can contribute to a healthier, more balanced lifestyle. Individuals often report sustained reductions in pain and stress levels, improved sleep patterns, and a greater sense of emotional resilience. The therapy's focus on holistic healing ensures that all aspects of a person's well-being are addressed, promoting long-term health and vitality.

In summary, Watsu therapy offers a comprehensive approach to health and well-being, with significant physical, mental, and emotional benefits. Through real-life examples and long-term effects, it is evident that Watsu can play a vital role in enhancing quality of life and supporting sustained health improvements.

CHAPTER FIVE

PREPARING FOR A WATSU THERAPY SESSION

Pre-Session Guidelines: What To Do Before Your Session

Before heading to your Watsu therapy session, it's essential to prepare your body and mind to ensure you get the most out of the experience. Hydrate well throughout the day, as staying hydrated can help your muscles relax more effectively during the session.

Avoid eating a heavy meal right before your appointment; instead, opt for a light snack if you're hungry. This prevents any discomfort during the floating and stretching movements of Watsu therapy.

Mentally, take a few moments to calm your mind. Practice deep breathing exercises or a short meditation to help you enter the session with a relaxed mindset. This mental preparation can make a significant difference in how you experience the therapy, allowing you to be more present and receptive to its benefits.

What To Wear: Appropriate Attire For Therapy

Choosing the right attire for your Watsu therapy session is crucial for your comfort and ease of movement. A well-fitted swimsuit is ideal, as it allows for a free range of motion while ensuring modesty. Women might prefer a one-piece swimsuit, while men can opt for swim trunks or briefs. Avoid swimsuits with excessive straps or decorations that could get in the way or cause discomfort.

Additionally, remove any jewelry or accessories before the session to prevent them from snagging or causing any interruptions. If you have long hair, tie it back or use a swim cap to keep it out of the way. This helps both you and your therapist focus on the therapy without distractions.

Setting Expectations: What You Should Expect During Your Session

Understanding what to expect during your Watsu therapy session can help you feel more at ease and open to the experience. Watsu therapy typically takes place in a warm pool, with the water temperature around 35°C (95°F). The warm water supports your body, allowing you to float effortlessly while your therapist gently moves, stretches, and massages you.

During the session, expect a combination of gentle rocking, stretches, and massage techniques. The movements are slow and rhythmic, designed to relax your muscles and mind. Some people might feel a deep sense of relaxation or even fall asleep during the session, which is perfectly normal. Communicate with your therapist about your comfort levels and any areas of tension or discomfort so they can adjust their techniques accordingly.

Communication With Your Therapist: How To Discuss Your Needs And Concerns

Effective communication with your Watsu therapist is key to a successful and beneficial session. Before the therapy begins, take a few minutes to discuss any specific needs or concerns you may have. Let your therapist know about any medical conditions, injuries, or areas of pain that they should be aware of. This information allows them to tailor the session to your unique needs and ensure your safety and comfort.

During the session, don't hesitate to speak up if you experience any discomfort or if you feel the need to adjust any part of the therapy. Your therapist is there to help you, and open communication ensures that the session remains beneficial and enjoyable for you. After the session, provide feedback about what worked well and what could be improved for future sessions.

Post-Session Care: Tips For After Your Session To Maximize Benefits

Taking care of yourself after a Watsu therapy session can enhance and prolong the benefits you experience. Once the session is over, take a few moments to slowly transition out of the pool. Allow yourself to sit quietly and absorb the relaxation you just experienced. Hydrate well by drinking plenty of water to help flush out any toxins released during the therapy.

Rest is important after a Watsu session. If possible, avoid strenuous activities for the rest of the day and allow your body to fully integrate the relaxation and stretches from the therapy. Gentle stretching or a light walk can help maintain a sense of relaxation and flexibility.

Listening to your body is crucial. Pay attention to how you feel and permit yourself to rest if needed. Some people might feel deeply relaxed, while others may experience a surge of energy. Both responses are normal and indicate that your body is processing the therapy in its way.

CHAPTER SIX

WATSU THERAPY FOR SPECIFIC CONDITIONS

Chronic Pain: How Watsu Can Help With Chronic Pain Management

Watsu therapy, a gentle form of bodywork performed in warm water, can be a powerful tool in managing chronic pain.

The buoyancy provided by the water reduces the strain on muscles and joints, allowing for pain-free movement and relaxation.

This environment enables the therapist to perform stretches and movements that might be difficult or impossible on land, targeting areas of tension and discomfort with ease.

For individuals suffering from conditions such as fibromyalgia, arthritis, or back pain, Watsu can significantly alleviate pain. The warm water helps to soothe muscles and improve blood circulation, which can reduce inflammation and promote healing.

Additionally, the gentle rocking and stretching movements used in Watsu therapy can release endorphins, the body's natural painkillers, providing immediate relief and promoting a sense of well-being.

Patients often report a decrease in pain levels following a Watsu session, as well as improved flexibility and range of motion.

The reduction in pain and tension can also lead to better sleep and a greater ability to engage in daily activities. By incorporating regular Watsu sessions into a chronic pain management plan, individuals can experience a holistic improvement in their overall quality of life.

Stress And Anxiety: Using Watsu To Manage Stress And Anxiety

Watsu therapy offers a unique and effective approach to managing stress and anxiety. The combination of warm water, gentle movement, and supportive touch creates a deeply relaxing experience that can significantly reduce stress levels. The warmth of the water helps to calm the nervous system, while the floating sensation promotes a sense of weightlessness and freedom from tension.

During a Watsu session, the therapist guides the client through a series of gentle stretches and movements, often accompanied by slow, rhythmic breathing. This mindful focus on the body and breath helps to quiet the mind and release mental and emotional stress. The soothing environment allows clients to let go of their worries and fully immerse themselves in the present moment.

Regular Watsu therapy can lead to lasting benefits for those struggling with anxiety. The deep relaxation achieved during sessions can help to lower cortisol levels, the body's primary stress hormone, and promote a sense of calm and balance. Many clients find that their anxiety symptoms decrease over time, and they are better able to cope with stressful situations in their daily lives.

Rehabilitation: Watsu's Role In Physical Rehabilitation

Watsu therapy can play a significant role in physical rehabilitation, offering a supportive and nurturing environment for recovery. The buoyancy of the water reduces the weight-bearing load on the body, making it easier for individuals to move and perform exercises without pain or strain. This makes Watsu an excellent option for those recovering from surgery, injury, or chronic conditions that limit mobility.

The therapist can use the water's resistance to create a customized exercise program tailored to the individual's needs. Gentle stretches, joint mobilizations, and muscle-strengthening exercises can be performed with greater ease in the water, enhancing the rehabilitation process. The warm water also promotes relaxation and increases blood flow to injured areas, accelerating healing and reducing inflammation.

Watsu therapy can be particularly beneficial for individuals with conditions such as spinal cord injuries, stroke, or traumatic brain injuries. The supportive environment allows for the gradual reintroduction of movement and the rebuilding of strength and coordination. Patients often report improved mobility, reduced pain, and enhanced overall function following regular Watsu sessions.

Pregnancy: Safe Practices And Benefits For Pregnant Individuals

Watsu therapy is a safe and beneficial practice for pregnant individuals, offering a unique way to relax and prepare for childbirth. The warm water provides a sense of weightlessness, reducing the pressure on the joints and spine that often accompanies pregnancy. This can alleviate common discomforts such as back pain, sciatica, and swelling in the legs and feet.

During a Watsu session, the therapist uses gentle movements and stretches to help relieve tension and improve circulation. The floating sensation and rhythmic movements can also promote relaxation and reduce stress, which is particularly important during pregnancy. Watsu therapy encourages deep breathing and mindfulness, helping to create a sense of calm and connection with the baby.

Safety is a primary concern when providing Watsu therapy to pregnant clients. The therapist ensures that all movements are gentle and supportive, avoiding any positions or stretches that could cause discomfort or harm.

Watsu can be adapted to each stage of pregnancy, with the therapist adjusting the techniques to accommodate the changing needs of the mother-to-be.

Regular Watsu sessions can help pregnant individuals maintain physical and emotional well-being throughout their pregnancy. The relaxation and stress relief provided by Watsu can lead to better sleep, reduced anxiety, and a greater sense of overall health. Many expectant mothers find that Watsu helps them to feel more prepared and confident as they approach childbirth.

Elderly Care: Adapting Watsu For Senior Clients

Watsu therapy can be highly beneficial for elderly clients, offering a gentle and effective way to maintain physical and emotional health. The warm water environment reduces the risk of injury and provides a safe space for seniors to engage in physical activity.

The buoyancy of the water supports the body, allowing for greater freedom of movement and reducing the strain on joints and muscles.

For seniors, Watsu therapy can improve flexibility, balance, and strength, helping to maintain mobility and independence. The therapist can tailor the session to the individual's needs, focusing on gentle stretches and movements that promote joint health and muscle function.

The warm water also helps to soothe aches and pains, providing relief from conditions such as arthritis and osteoporosis.

In addition to the physical benefits, Watsu therapy can have a positive impact on mental and emotional well-being.

The relaxation and stress relief achieved during a Watsu session can help to reduce anxiety and depression, which are common concerns for many seniors. The supportive and nurturing environment also promotes a sense of connection and well-being, enhancing the overall quality of life.

Adapting Watsu therapy for elderly clients involves careful attention to their individual needs and limitations.

The therapist ensures that all movements are safe and comfortable, and may use additional supports or modifications as needed.

With regular Watsu sessions, seniors can enjoy improved physical health, greater relaxation, and a more positive outlook on life.

CHAPTER SEVEN

COMMON CONCERNS AND MISCONCEPTIONS

Safety Concerns: Addressing Common Fears And How To Ensure Safety

One of the primary concerns many people have about Watsu therapy is its safety. This concern is often rooted in the unfamiliarity with the therapy and its unique approach.

Watsu, which involves receiving therapeutic movements and stretches while floating in warm water, may seem daunting at first. However, it is essential to understand that Watsu therapy is designed with safety in mind.

The water's warmth and buoyancy help reduce strain on the body, making it a gentle, low-impact therapy.

To ensure safety during a Watsu session, it is crucial to communicate openly with your therapist about any health issues or concerns.

 A qualified Watsu therapist will conduct a thorough assessment before beginning the session and will tailor the therapy to suit your individual needs.

They are trained to handle various physical conditions and to make adjustments as necessary to ensure your comfort and safety.

Additionally, the water temperature is carefully regulated to avoid overheating or discomfort. By following these guidelines and maintaining an open dialogue with your therapist, you can enjoy a safe and beneficial Watsu experience.

Effectiveness Doubts: Addressing Skepticism About Therapy Benefits

Skepticism about the effectiveness of Watsu therapy is not uncommon. Some people may question whether floating and gentle movements can truly provide significant benefits. It's important to understand that Watsu therapy is supported by both anecdotal evidence and clinical studies. Many individuals report feeling profound relaxation, relief from muscle tension, and improved range of motion after Watsu sessions.

Watsu therapy's effectiveness stems from its ability to combine the soothing effects of water with therapeutic movements. The warm water reduces muscle tension and promotes relaxation, while the therapist's gentle stretches and movements help to release deep-seated tension and improve flexibility. While results can vary from person to person, many find that regular Watsu sessions lead to noticeable improvements in their physical and emotional well-being. If you're skeptical, consider starting with a trial session to experience the benefits firsthand.

Misconceptions About Water Therapy: Clarifying Common Misunderstandings

Water therapy, including Watsu, is often surrounded by misconceptions. One common misunderstanding is that it is simply a form of relaxation or a luxury treatment rather than a legitimate therapeutic approach. In reality, Watsu therapy is a recognized method of addressing physical and emotional issues through the unique properties of water. It integrates principles from traditional massage and movement therapies to provide a holistic treatment experience.

Another misconception is that water therapy is only suitable for those who are already in good health.

On the contrary, Watsu therapy can benefit individuals with various physical conditions, including chronic pain, stress, and mobility issues.

The buoyancy of the water supports the body, making it easier to perform movements that might be challenging on land. Watsu therapy is adaptable and can be customized to meet the needs of individuals with different health conditions.

Cost And Accessibility: Discussing Costs And Finding Affordable Options

Cost can be a significant concern when considering Watsu therapy. Prices for Watsu sessions can vary depending on location, therapist expertise, and session length. In general, Watsu therapy may be more expensive than other forms of massage or physical therapy due to the specialized training of the therapists and the use of a dedicated therapy pool.

However, there are ways to make Watsu therapy more accessible. Some therapists offer sliding scale fees or package deals, which can reduce the cost per session if you commit to multiple sessions.

Additionally, certain wellness centers or clinics might offer Watsu therapy as part of a broader range of services, potentially making it more affordable.

It's also worth checking with local health insurance providers to see if they offer any coverage for complementary therapies like

Watsu. Exploring these options can help you find a solution that fits your budget.

Finding Qualified Therapists: How To Choose A Skilled Watsu Therapist

Choosing a qualified Watsu therapist is crucial for a positive therapy experience. A skilled therapist will have completed specialized training in Watsu and will have experience working with a variety of clients. When searching for a therapist, look for credentials and certifications from reputable organizations, such as the Watsu International Association or similar bodies.

It's also important to consider the therapist's experience and approach. A good Watsu therapist should be able to provide references or testimonials from previous clients.

Additionally, scheduling a consultation or trial session can help you assess the therapist's compatibility with your needs and preferences. During this initial meeting, discuss any health concerns and ask about their approach to therapy to ensure that it aligns with your goals. By taking these steps, you can find a qualified Watsu therapist who will provide a safe and effective therapeutic experience.

CHAPTER EIGHT

FAQS ABOUT WATSU THERAPY

What Should I Expect In My First Session?

Your first Watsu therapy session is designed to be a gentle and relaxing introduction to this unique form of aquatic bodywork.

When you arrive at the therapy pool, you'll be greeted by your therapist, who will explain the process and answer any initial questions you might have. The pool is typically warm, around 35°C (95°F), which helps to relax your muscles and promote a sense of calm.

You'll start by floating in the water, supported by your therapist. They will guide you through a series of movements and stretches, using the water's buoyancy to facilitate gentle joint mobilizations and muscle stretches. This allows for a greater range of motion than what is typically possible on land. You might experience a sense of weightlessness and deep relaxation as you float, which is a hallmark of Watsu therapy.

It's common to feel a bit uncertain at first, especially if you're not used to being in water or receiving bodywork. However, your therapist will move slowly and carefully, ensuring you feel comfortable and supported throughout the session. Communication is key, so don't hesitate to express any concerns or ask questions during the process.

How Often Should I Have Watsu Therapy?

The frequency of Watsu therapy sessions can vary based on individual needs and goals. For general relaxation and stress relief, many people find that a session once or twice a month is sufficient. If you are dealing with specific physical issues, such as chronic pain or recovery from an injury, your therapist might recommend more frequent sessions, perhaps weekly or bi-weekly.

It's important to listen to your body and communicate with your therapist about how you're feeling between sessions. They can help you adjust the frequency based on your progress and any changes in your condition. Over time, as your body adapts and heals, the number of sessions might decrease.

Are There Any Side Effects?

Watsu therapy is generally considered very safe, but like any therapeutic intervention, it can have some side effects. The most common side effects are mild and temporary, such as feeling tired or slightly sore after a session.

This is typically a result of your muscles and joints being stretched and moved in new ways.

In rare cases, some individuals might experience dizziness or nausea, particularly if they are sensitive to motion or have been in warm water for an extended period. If you experience these symptoms, it's important to inform your therapist immediately. They can adjust the intensity and duration of the session to ensure your comfort.

To minimize side effects, make sure to stay hydrated before and after your session, and avoid eating a heavy meal right before. Additionally, if you have any pre-existing medical conditions, discuss them with your therapist beforehand to tailor the session to your specific needs.

Can Watsu Therapy Be Combined With Other Treatments?

Watsu therapy can be an excellent complement to other forms of treatment, both conventional and alternative. Many people use it alongside physical therapy, chiropractic care, massage, and even psychotherapy. The gentle, supportive nature of Watsu makes it a versatile addition to a comprehensive treatment plan.

When combined with physical therapy, Watsu can help to enhance mobility and flexibility, making land-based exercises easier to perform. For those undergoing chiropractic care, Watsu can relax muscles and reduce tension, potentially improving the effectiveness of adjustments.

It's important to coordinate with all your healthcare providers when combining treatments. Make sure each practitioner is aware of the other therapies you are receiving so they can tailor their approach accordingly. This integrated approach ensures that all aspects of your health and wellness are addressed harmoniously.

How Do I Find A Qualified Therapist?

Finding a qualified Watsu therapist is crucial to ensuring a safe and effective experience. Start by looking for practitioners who are certified by reputable organizations such as the Worldwide Aquatic Bodywork Association (WABA). Certification ensures that the therapist has undergone rigorous training and adheres to professional standards.

You can also ask for recommendations from your healthcare providers, friends, or family members who have experienced Watsu therapy. Personal referrals can often lead you to highly skilled and reputable therapists.

When you contact a potential therapist, ask about their training, experience, and approach to Watsu therapy. It's also a good idea to schedule a preliminary meeting or phone call to discuss your goals and any specific needs or concerns you might have. This initial conversation can help you determine if the therapist is a good fit for you.

Lastly, trust your instincts. A good Watsu therapist should make you feel comfortable, respected, and supported. If you feel at ease with them, you're more likely to have a positive and beneficial experience.

CHAPTER NINE

RESOURCES AND FURTHER READING

Books And Articles: Recommended Reading Materials On Watsu Therapy

For those looking to delve deeper into Watsu therapy, a range of books and articles offer comprehensive insights into its techniques, benefits, and applications.

Books such as "Watsu: Freeing the Body in Water" by Harold Dull provide foundational knowledge and detailed explanations of the various movements and their therapeutic effects.

Another highly recommended book is "Aquatic Therapy Using Watsu®: Basic and Advanced Techniques," which caters to both beginners and advanced practitioners.

Academic articles in journals such as the Journal of Bodywork and Movement Therapies also offer peer-reviewed research on the efficacy of Watsu in different therapeutic contexts. Reading these materials can provide a solid theoretical background and enhance practical understanding.

Online Resources: Websites And Online Communities For Further Learning

The internet hosts a wealth of information on Watsu therapy, with several dedicated websites and online communities where enthusiasts and practitioners can share knowledge and experiences. Websites like Watsu.com offer extensive resources, including articles, videos, and forums where users can discuss techniques and benefits. Social media platforms also have active groups and pages where members post instructional videos, personal experiences, and updates on the latest research in the field. Participating in these online communities can be incredibly beneficial for continuous learning and staying updated with new developments in Watsu therapy.

Professional Organizations: Key Organizations Related To Watsu Therapy

Several professional organizations are dedicated to the practice and promotion of Watsu therapy. The Worldwide Aquatic Bodywork Association (WABA) is one of the most prominent, providing resources, certification programs, and a global network of practitioners. Another notable organization is the International Watsu Association, which supports the professional development of Watsu therapists and promotes high standards of practice. These organizations often host conferences, workshops, and seminars, providing opportunities for professional growth and networking. Joining these organizations can provide access to valuable resources and a supportive community of fellow practitioners.

Workshops And Training: Opportunities For Hands-On Learning And Certification

Hands-on training is crucial for mastering Watsu therapy, and numerous workshops and training programs are available for those interested in becoming certified practitioners. These workshops range from introductory courses to advanced certification programs and are often conducted by experienced practitioners. Training programs typically include both theoretical and practical components, ensuring that participants gain a comprehensive understanding of Watsu techniques and principles. Attending these workshops not only enhances practical skills but also provides opportunities to receive feedback from experienced therapists and to practice in a supportive environment.

Contact Information: How To Connect With Watsu Therapy Professionals And Organizations

Connecting with Watsu therapy professionals and organizations can be a vital step for anyone looking to learn more about this therapeutic practice or seeking professional guidance. Most professional organizations, such as WABA and the International Watsu Association, have contact details listed on their websites, including email addresses and phone numbers. Additionally, many individual practitioners have personal websites or social media profiles where they can be contacted for appointments or inquiries. Networking with professionals in the field can provide personalized advice, mentorship opportunities, and information on local Watsu sessions or workshops.

By leveraging these resources, aspiring Watsu therapists can build a solid foundation of knowledge and skills, while those already practicing can continue to grow and refine their techniques. Engaging with books, online communities, professional organizations, and hands-on training opportunities ensures a well-rounded and comprehensive approach to learning and practicing Watsu therapy.